Table of Contents

Comparison of Addison's Disease and Cushing's Syndrome: Symptoms, Causes, and Treatment

1. Introduction

Addison's disease and Cushing's syndrome are two of the illnesses manifested with symptoms attributable to the final consequences of adrenocortical hormone hyperfunction and hypofunction. The similarity of the adverse events prevents the use of these symptoms as tools for a differential diagnosis. Addison's disease may need to take one or more of these medications: prednisone, aldosterone replacements, antifungal medication, and surgery may be recommended. Education and long-term treatment with a dietician, treatment for other health problems, and managing stress are also important. The treatments for Cushing's syndrome include surgery, radiation, cortisol-inhibiting drugs, treatments for health problems caused by Cushing's syndrome, and treatment may be necessary for other health problems caused by Cushing's syndrome.

Addison's disease and Cushing's syndrome are both characterized by a dysfunction of the endocrine system. Addison's disease, also referred to as primary adrenal insufficiency or adrenocortical hypofunction, is characterized by a decrease or cessation of the production of adrenocortical hormones, while Cushing's syndrome is a condition of hypercortisolism. Addison's disease occurs due to insufficient levels of cortisol and possibly aldosterone, allowing increased levels of adrenocorticotropic hormone (ACTH), while Cushing's syndrome arises due to excessive production of cortisol stimulating syndrome of hypercortisolism. This essay will briefly discuss the symptoms for the pair of diseases and its corresponding medications and treatments.

2. Understanding Endocrine Disorders

The endocrine system is composed of glands and organs in the body that secrete hormones. These hormones are essential for proper body functions that include metabolism, growth, and the body's response to stimuli, stress, and injury. When these hormone-secreting glands and organs are affected by disease or produce too many (or too little) hormones, many aspects of health and daily functioning can be impacted. There are many endocrine disorders relating to the various glands and hormones present in the body, including sex hormones, thyroid hormone, hormone regulating blood sugar, hormone regulating mineral balance, and hormones that modulate salt and water balance. This document will only encompass two endocrine disorders, Addison's Disease and Cushing's Syndrome, focusing on background, symptoms, causes, diagnosis, and treatment.

Endocrine disorders involve problems with the body's hormone-secreting glands and organs, called endocrine glands. One such condition is Addison's Disease, which is characterized by damage to the adrenal gland. This results in the lack of production of cortisol (stress hormone) and aldosterone (a hormone associated with mineral and electrolyte regulation), which can manifest in many symptoms. At the other end of the spectrum is Cushing's Syndrome, a disorder characterized by an excessive production of cortisol in the body. This can be the result of overmedication with steroidal hormones or the overproduction of adrenocorticotropic hormone (ACTH) that causes the excess cortisol production. This condition is also characterized by many symptoms and can lead to serious health implications when left untreated. Inadequate cortisol is harmful for the body, as is excessive cortisol. Proper hormone production and regulation is crucial for maintaining a healthy equilibrium within the body.

2.1. Overview of Addison's Disease and Cushing's Syndrome

This chapter gives an overview of the two disorders, followed by a detailed study of symptoms, causes, tests and diagnosis, treatment, screening, risk factors, living with, complications, etc. of Addison's disease and Cushing's syndrome. It is desirable that the book would be useful for physicians, nurses, healthcare professionals, endocrinologists, neurologists, and experts dealing with clinical cases and research. The chapter may also be beneficial for students, educators, physicians, researchers, academics, or anyone looking for deeper insights into adrenal-related hormones in the body and the complications or disorders associated with them.

Both Addison's disease and Cushing's syndrome are two of the several rare disorders that could occur in the endocrine system. Whereas Addison's disease results from the destruction of the adrenal cortex, Cushing's syndrome occurs when there is cortisol excess in the body resulting from overproduction of cortisol by one or both of the adrenal glands. Patients can also develop it due to the consumption of exogenous glucocorticoids such as prednisolone, dexamethasone, etc.

3. Symptoms of Addison's Disease and Cushing's Syndrome

3.1. General Symptoms

3.2. Specific Symptoms

4. Causes of Addison's Disease and Cushing's Syndrome

The listed primary and secondary causes of Addison's disease are rather similar to those found in the cases of Cushing's syndrome. The latter condition may also be developed due to an incorrect taking of artificial hormones that the patients use during their life routine. In other cases, men and women can develop Cushing's syndrome while taking corticosteroid hormones for other health problems. When it comes to the treatment of Addison's disease or Cushing's syndrome, there is still no cure for the syndromes. At the same time, the conditions may be treated both with medicines and surgery. The patients must use the treatment exactly as their doctor prescribes.

Addison's disease can affect a person due to different causes. The most common cause of Addison's disease is the genetic predisposition of a person to develop the disease. Doctors state that about 90% of patients have positive relatives with symptoms of the condition. Speaking of Addison's disease, both men and women have the same risk of developing it. Today, the syndrome is also primarily developed due to the patient's own body attacking itself. Scientists are likely to be on the way to determine the exact cause of Addison's disease. At the same time, Cushing's syndrome, as Addison's disease, occurs due to various conditions. Almost the same reasons that are present in the case of the Addison's disease are common in cases of

Cushing's syndrome: heredity, age, and the tendency of the inner body to attack itself.

4.1. Primary Causes

4.2.2.a. Adrenal Adenoma can cause primary causes of Cushing's Syndrome and is the least aggressive of the two types. Adrenal Carcinoma is primary causes of Cushing's Syndrome and are rare, aggressive as malignant and tend to metastasize quickly. If they are producing hormones, they generally cause Cushing's Syndrome before they are discovered, making prompt surgical treatment necessary.

4.2.2. Cushing's Syndrome, on the other hand, is caused by an overactive adrenal cortex, usually due to the administration of excess glucocorticoid medication. Cushing's Syndrome can occur from this chronic exposure to excess glucocorticoids, most commonly secondary to exogenous steroid use because of an autoimmune response of the patient's own adrenal tissues. It can also be caused by a primary adrenal tumor, pituitary tumor that secretes ACTH (adrenocorticotropic hormone), or an ACTH-secreting tumor that likely originates outside the pituitary. This last cause is called ectopic Cushing's Syndrome, or ectopic Cushing's Disease.

4.2.1. Addison's Disease, or primary adrenal insufficiency, is caused by the progressive destruction of the adrenal cortex, most commonly due to an autoimmune response. Some other causes include infections, infarctions, tumors, metastases, hemorrhage, certain genetic defects, and the use of certain medications. However, many cases of Addison's Disease remain idiopathic. Around 70% of the adrenal cortex is already destroyed by the time symptoms become noticeable.

4.1. Primary causes.

4.2. Secondary Causes

The first case was published 100 years ago by Katz and Eisenkraft in 1926. More than 500 cases were diagnosed by 1958. In the past, dating before contemporary knowledge, granulomatous etiology was the primary cause of patients seen in outpatient units. Nowadays, patients who are generally more asymptomatic and have a physical examination that is largely preview come to the attention of clinics. Since the history of granulomatous disorder is inquired into, these all are candidates. Buie diseases of the skin - most commonly lupus pernio and ulcerated nodules of the extremities, hypercalcemia and/or increased calciuria, hypophosphatemia or high levels of serum alkaline phosphatase, increased urea nitrogen and plasma creatinine, and emptying disorders.

The next largest category of 17 secondary causes (29.8%) consists of those associated with an immune condition, either rheumatoid arthritis, ankylosing spondylitis, or Sjogren's syndrome; but this is not nearly so overwhelming a picture. Nor is the presence of a secondary cause always associated with PRO's refusal. Overall, in 4 secondary-cause cases of this sample, PRO refused. In 2 cases brought by incompetents, PRO has no obvious refusal, but it is material to observe that PPP has not, for that matter, supported the application. The hormonal syndromes of Addison's disease and diuretic-dependent y-phase primary aldosteronism bring together cortisol-producing adrenal pathology and the unexpected persistence of places cells secreting y cortisol. Studies exploring the cognitive impacts of yCs in these hypercortisol series indicate impairments that are more marked in PDAC than in primary hyperaldosteronism HAsucNEW and Cushing's syndrome.

2. Addison's Disease and Cushing's Syndrome

5. Diagnosis and Differential Diagnosis

In winter times or in case of altered pigment distribution, leading to the patient's attention towards the skin, positron emission tomography (PET) or a computed tomography (CT) scan may provide evidence of a hormone-producing adrenal tumor or other pathological lesions of the adrenal glands or the pituitary. A classification difference can be made between primary and secondary active Cushing's syndrome. Recently, the first screening methods regarding an endogenous Cushing's syndrome have been established. The diagnostic differentiation with the exclusion of a pseudo-CS is considered as the key point of laboratory diagnosis for se-Cortisol (T) determination.

Diagnosis processes. Often, a healthcare provider diagnoses individual people affected by AC based on their medical history, symptoms, and physical examination. Physical examination, in combination with an evaluation of adrenal function, confirms the disease. The highly increased UFC excretion, which is independent of the circadian rhythm, is typical for CS. High levels of ACTH with cortisol levels below the normal range are characteristic for AD or primary adrenal insufficiency, in contrast. As a diagnostic tool, X-ray and ultrasound can be helpful in the course of the differential diagnostics process.

5.1. Diagnostic Tests

The low dose Synacthen test (LDT) is quick and convenient and requires no specific clinician training for its procedure, but is not universally available because of Synacthen's limited use and availability and potential problems with storage. Using a long-acting form of synthetic ACTH as an alternative and comparing it with Inferior Advancement, a simple and practical method with excellent cl...

Diagnostic tests for adrenocortical insufficiency include the measurement of basal ACTH and cortisol levels, or the use of a screening test to replace these measurements. Contrary to common belief, synacthen (tetracosactid; synthetic ACTH(1-24)) is not currently available as a registered product in many countries, including the UK. Cortrosyn has been the product of choice for the assessment of adrenal glands, but it is no longer available. An alternative agent, Synacthen Depot, was shown to be better than Cortrosyn and is used in many countries. In 2018, the FDA approved Hydrocortisone Sodium Succinate in a 250 mcg dose vial. The EDMONT MCG edition is being verified for its efficiency in study conditions and may replace Synacthen in the near future, but it is currently only recommended for the Glucagon Stimulation Test.

Once the clinical presentation has given rise to a suspicion of the underlying condition, diagnostic tests are needed to confirm or exclude the diagnosis. The natural history of Addison's disease is one of progressive deterioration, and it is important that the disease is diagnosed and treated adequately as soon as possible to prevent any morbidity. As outlined above, patients with adrenal insufficiency usually present with non-specific complaints. Although no clinical trial has been performed, one can assume that the increase in morbidity is associated with the delay in diagnosis if the disease is not diagnosed 'early' and treated adequately.

5.2. Differentiating Between Addison's Disease and Cushing's Syndrome

Furthermore, both diseases can be presented with primary, secondary, and tertiary forms. In the primary form of Addison's disease, high plasma adrenocorticotropic hormone (ACTH) levels together with low cortisol values suggest the disease. In the primary form of Cushing's syndrome, high urinary free cortisol (UFC)/creatinine (c) values together with high ACTH levels should be detected. The differential diagnosis between secondary and tertiary forms of both diseases is based on using the CRH test and measuring plasma concentration of ACTH. Although MRI of the pituitary gland shows the tumor or the microadenoma in positive patients, the image of the tumor might not be seen in the early period of the disease and surgery will not be enhanced. Patients with negative MRI results can be managed as patients with the primary disease management-wise.

Addison's disease is suggested when the symptoms include weight reduction, hypotension, generalized brownish pigmentation of the skin, and anorexia together, or when cortisol-related metabolites are low or within the normal limits. Cushing's syndrome is suggested when the symptoms include weight increase, diabetes, easy bruising, and a round face, especially with buffalo hump, together, and cortisol-related metabolites are within the normal limits.

When diagnosing a disorder, not only should any disorder with similar characteristics be distinguished from it, but also the possibility of it being caused by a different disease. Addison's disease and Cushing's syndrome are both endocrine diseases related to cortical hormones of the adrenal gland. The signs and symptoms have similarities and can be observed in various combinations according to the severity of the diseases, which may make differentiation difficult.

6. Treatment Options

Addison's disease and Cushing's syndrome may both be thoroughly treated. Your medical care staff will assist you in determining which treatment is best for you as an individual. Addison's disease is often treated with a steroid replacement medication. There are numerous drugs available that contain this synthetic hormone, and people with the disorder can work with their doctor to select the one which is best suited to their requirements. Because it has a fast-acting hormone, hydrocortisone is frequently recommended. In numerous instances, extra mineralocorticoid medications may be prescribed in order to better manage the symptoms. Although these medications are very effective, your pulse and blood pressure need to be checked on a regular basis so that the appropriate dosage can be determined.

Cushing's syndrome may be either an illness on its own or a side effect of another illness. In all cases, the first step to healing involves treating the condition that produced the excess cortisol in the first place. Depending on the source of the dilemma, this may require medication, surgery, or radiation therapy. When a single medication does not control the cortisol levels, a mixture of drugs may be prescribed. Treatment for Cushing's syndrome, on the other hand, will be tailored to each patient.

Addison's disease is usually treated using a steroid replacement medication. Several medications contain this artificial hormone, and people with the disorder can work with their practitioner to find the one that best suits their requirements.

Addison's disease and Cushing's syndrome can both be effectively treated. The medical professionals on your treatment team will work with you to decide which form of treatment is best suited to your specific situation.

6.1. Medications

Similarly, the approach to treating Cushing's depends on the reason for the excessive levels of cortisol. However, if the problem lies with the pituitary or adrenal glands, treating the underlying cause is generally the primary approach. Often, this can be done using medications. However, if the issue is with a benign tumor, surgery may be the best option. Regardless of the underlying cause, the main goal of treating Cushing's syndrome is generally to lower cortisol by reducing its production in the body.

People with Addison's disease have to supplement the hormones their adrenal glands are no longer producing. Cortisol is replaced orally through tablets that need to be taken two to three times a day. One of the following three medications is generally prescribed to replace aldosterone, which acts to control sodium and potassium balance in the body: Fludrocortisone (Florinef) - The most common medication used to treat Addison's disease. Fludrocortisone acetate (titration compounding pharmacy cream) - The preferred route of administration, which makes it easier to adjust the dose. Percorten, naturally derived desoxycorticosterone pivalate - Helps regulate electrolytes and fluid. Sometimes, with Addison's disease, patients are also given short-acting glucocorticoids to take during times of stress.

6.2. Surgery

If surgery is not possible, alternative treatments include daily intake of corticosteroid tablets, possibly along with additional medications. There is no one-size-fits-all treatment regimen. In addition, as some of these diseases present with severe depression, there may be some hesitation in treating them at all unless their mental health is improved. The mental problems that develop as a result of these conditions are often mistakenly treated first, rather than ensuring effective control over the endocrinopathy.

As is the case for Addison's disease, surgery may also be employed as a treatment regimen for Cushing's syndrome, although the primary consideration will be to maintain homeostasis of body level cortisol. The aim of surgical excision is to remove the tumor (if present) that is generating ACTH-secreting tumors are typically located in the pituitary gland. Once resected, the release of cortisol will cease thus returning the HPA to its normal functional capacity. The dentist should be aware that some patients will still require HRT following excision, and that healing will be slowed and anti-inflammatory medications may be required.

Yes, surgery may be performed as a treatment regimen for Addison's disease. Given the recent changes in treatment of the endocrinopathy, this approach is now considered rare. Current practices have moved towards chronic supplementation via corticosteroid tablets. The dentist should be aware that the patient may still require HRT postoperatively.

6.3. Lifestyle and Home Remedies

- Proper nutrition: Low blood sugar can lead to dizziness, shaky hands, and fainting. By adjusting your diet and eating frequently, your blood sugar can stabilize. - Lower stress: This may require some lifestyle adjustments, but by minimizing stress, you may be less prone to severe fatigue and digestive upset. - Cushing's syndrome treatment of underlying condition: Lifestyle and home remedies can be used to treat any underlying conditions at the source. To avoid taking in too much sodium, limit your salt intake. You'll probably need follow-up visits with your healthcare provider to monitor your condition if you've recently had surgery to remove a pituitary tumor or adrenal gland. Include regular check-ins with your healthcare provider, they have a better idea of your specific conditions. These appointments can help keep track of the effectiveness of the treatments you are using, help to anticipate or mitigate the side effects of treatments, and offer the opportunity to check for evidence of recurrence.

Your healthcare provider will likely provide you with an oral corticosteroid medication to replace the steroidal hormones your body can no longer produce on its own. They'll probably also prescribe regular blood tests to see if you're responding well. In the meantime, there are some lifestyle adjustments that you can make to help ease the symptoms of Addison's disease.

7. Prognosis and Complications

Complications of Addison's disease and Cushing's syndrome Addison's disease and Cushing's syndrome can cause many complications. Addison's disease can lead to an Addisonian crisis, causing an abrupt onset of severe symptoms. This is a serious and life-threatening condition that requires hospitalization. Cushing's syndrome can cause weakened bone density leading to osteoporosis and fractures. Due to an increased risk of developing hyperglycemia or Type 2 diabetes mellitus, it can also affect metabolism and blood sugar levels. Elevated blood pressure and weight gain are associated with the increased risk of developing adverse cardiac events. Heat intolerance, muscle weakness, fatigue, and tender bones can also be caused by Cushing's syndrome.

Prognosis of Addison's disease and Cushing's syndrome Addison's disease (primary adrenal insufficiency) is a chronic endocrine disorder. It is a lifelong illness; however, with lifelong steroid hormone replacement treatment, it can be effectively controlled. Cushing's syndrome is also a chronic disorder. Prognosis varies based on the underlying cause and success of treatment. Some studies suggest that treating the syndrome may decrease the associated cardiovascular mortality, but other studies suggest the opposite. Adrenal tumors have a higher chance of cancer or becoming cancerous when they are larger than 10 cm.

7.1. Outlook for Addison's Disease and Cushing's Syndrome Patients

A handful of people with Addison's disease require a hospital emergency room visit to manage it. There is a rather good prognosis for those who are not affected by chronic adrenal insufficiency, i.e., the prognosis that symptoms and signs will resolve. Symptoms of Cushing's syndrome are generally reversible and clear up once the problem has been treated or resolved. Following appropriate treatment or surgery, most Cushing's syndrome patients can expect quick recovery and a good-quality life. If the problem causing the steroid excess is malignant, complications may occur during the treatment process. Restricted life expectancy and a poor prognosis are associated with malignant forms of adrenal cancer. Cushing's syndrome related to an ectopic and pituitary ACTH-producing tumor has an excellent long-term prognosis.

In summary, those with Addison's disease can lead a relatively normal life provided they adhere to treatment recommendations and lead a healthy lifestyle. The majority of Addison's disease patients have a normal lifespan without any significant disability. If not diagnosed or treated in time, the long-term prognosis of Addison's disease patients may be poor and symptoms may worsen and become more severe. Although this condition does not go away, it is possible for individuals to continue with normal activities.

7.2. Potential Complications

Cushing's syndrome is caused by an excess of corticosteroids and is a serious condition that often results in many fatal complications, including more than 50 diverse and potentially fatal disorders. It is associated with diagnosed diabetes. Hypertension (50-85%) is present in more than 80% of patients with Cushing's syndrome. Such hypertension can be devastating and is more severe and difficult to control than primary hypertension. Some risk factors have been identified as increasing the likelihood of an unsuccessful outcome in patients who are operated on. Although some complications cannot be treated and could result in a patient's death, others may be treatable or will go away once the illness has been treated.

Addison's disease is associated with risks such as fatigue due to muscle weakness, mood swings or cognitive slowing, hypotension, or darkening of the freckles of the body, among others. If unmedicated or poorly treated, an adrenal crisis or adrenal shock is a potential complication of chronic adrenal insufficiency. An adrenal crisis is one of the most challenging complications that a patient can face and always requires immediate treatment. The most common and fatal development of the disease occurs after a patient undergoes major surgery. Also, both psychological and physical stress and infection can lead to an adrenal crisis. Furthermore, hospitalized patients with an undiagnosed condition may suffer from an acute adrenal crisis. Addison's disease can affect a human being in several ways, both personally and professionally, alongside the mental stress of having to cope with chronic illness.

8. Prevention Strategies

Many people develop Cushing's syndrome or Addison's disease even though they have no known risk factors for the disease. Given the lack of known prevention strategies, the proactive strategies for these conditions are focused on individuals who are known to be at higher risk for developing disease. Early identification of Cushing's syndrome and Addison's disease allows for individuals to seek appropriate treatment from an endocrinologist when there are no or only mild symptoms. Scheduled follow-ups and cross-sectional imaging for individuals with a known adrenal tumor are also considered relatively cost-effective interventions that can help to identify early tumors that require medical treatment.

Currently, Addison's disease and Cushing's syndrome are generally well-recognized conditions with good treatment options. In addition, many individuals with the potential to develop these conditions are identified prior to the onset of symptoms, and specific preventative measures are available. Behavioral changes for prevention integrate stress reduction, weight loss, and reducing the consumption of alcohol and excessive caffeine. The use of exogenous corticosteroids for extended periods carries a potential risk of developing iatrogenic Cushing's syndrome. As the symptoms develop from the same hormone system in the body, individuals should be vigilant about the onset of new symptoms and should maintain follow-up with their healthcare provider.

9. Current Research and Future Directions

Some new types of diagnostic tools have been explored, but their specific worth has yet to be determined: CT laparoscopy with adrenocortical vein sampling, whole-genome DNA methylation profiling, and machine learning to differentiate between the different primary and secondary forms of adrenal insufficiency, and a 4-mg oral or intravenous (IV) Synacthen test to substantially reduce the number of assessments used at 1 mg. Four small studies used adrenal vein sampling for differentiating between unilateral and bilateral primary aldosteronism of the adrenal glands. Overall, patients should be treated at centres experienced in diagnosing, treating, and maintaining cortisol disorders. More studies on genetic testing in clinical practice for patients suspected of having adrenal insufficiency, whether primary or secondary, and more surveillance studies are needed. In addition, the potential long-term effects of prolonged glucocorticoid deficiency in patients who initially improved after removing the source of elevated or suppressed cortisol, and whether or not patients should continue to take lifelong glucocorticoid replacement therapy, should be discussed, according to these authors. Several researchers have initiated multi-centre, international, and national biological registries to gain a better understanding of the etiology, clinical evaluation, treatment, and long-term follow-up of patients with rare diseases such as Addison's disease and Cushing's syndrome.

Current research on Addison's and Cushing's diseases primarily focuses on developing new treatments, diagnostics, and predictive tools. In a systematic review of articles published in 2018, researchers reported a few potential innovative therapeutic strategies for treating both diseases, such as metyrapone and osilodrostat as adrenal-blocking agents, levoketoconazole and CORT125822 as dual 11b-hydroxylase and 17a-hydroxylase inhibitors, and pasireotide as a somatostatin analogue for treating patients with Cushing's disease, especially those who cannot be cured through surgery. Different imaging techniques and potential biomarkers have been studied to establish whether the adrenal glands function poorly following documented hypopituitarism, rather than relying on dynamic tests, the authors suggested.

Comparative Study of Addison's Disease and Cushing Syndrome

1. Introduction

Cushing syndrome is an uncommon clinical manifestation with symptoms that may be subclinical or may appear either late or at an advanced stage. It is caused by a rare disease of the pituitary. Survival rates increase when necessary preparation and prompt intervention are taken. The increased diagnosis and detection of Cushing's syndrome are due to advances in measurement methods, widespread access to refined MRI scans, regular visits to healthcare professionals and laboratory researchers, and low-dose tests for emergency use. A thorough and predictable focus is emerging.

Addison's disease, also known as primary adrenal insufficiency, is a rare and chronic disorder characterized by an unregulated lack of corticosteroids, mineralocorticoids, and other endocrine hormones as a result of a defect in the adrenal cortex itself. Cushing's syndrome, which is a potential cause of adrenal insufficiency, can be caused by both endogenous and exogenous glucocorticoids. It is diagnosed by an individual's ability to respond to the adrenal glands to overcome impaired physiological stress responses. Cushing's disease is responsible for mineralocorticoid and adrenal androgen deficit disorders, as the high amount of mineralocorticoids and glucocorticoids help to control feedback for regulating function in ACTH-secreting pituitary adenomas. The physiological causes of hypocortisolism that contribute to Addison's disease involve dysfunctions of glucocorticoids and ACTH-secreting pituitary adenomas that regulate ACTH and adrenal glands.

1.1. Background and Significance

It is important to analyze the functions of any endocrine hormone as it will help predict various pathological responses in other systems of the body. Interestingly, we could also predict the prognosis of the patients, marker diagnosis, treatment outcome, or the prompt to undergo surgery if diagnosed with any underlying pathological conditions. Literature studies have demonstrated that either adrenal insufficiency or oversecretion showed various mental health outcomes. Hormonal imbalances may also occur due to a median part of the response as a result of sequential diseases of the adrenals. Currently, many medical indications, especially in pediatrics, adrenal function analysis should be studied in a comparative manner with either a hyperactivity disorder or an inadequate activity of the adrenals. However, the main focus of this study would be a comparative one that includes the clinical and etiological comparison of Addison's disease and Cushing syndrome.

Endocrine system modifications can contribute to the onset of some mental health alterations. Studies have reported the impact of both hyper and hypo cortisol activity. The adverse effects, outcomes, and prediction of therapies, along with the comorbidities associated with Cushing patients, have been studied. It is of interest to study both the hyper and hypo functions of cortisol as a comparative study in the medical field. Cushing and Addison syndrome or disease may share many common physiological effects; therefore, we decided to conduct this review article to understand the comparative study of Addison's disease and Cushing syndrome, which involve the hyposecretion of cortisol hormone in the adrenals.

1.2. Purpose and Scope

Addison's disease and Cushing syndrome are similar because, in both, the negative feedback loop in cortisol (hydrocortisone) production fails. The primary distinctness in presentation stems from the different etiologies the diseases share, the one characterized by low hormone secretion (Addison's disease) and the other by high hormone secretion (Cushing syndrome). These endocrine disorders have features in common, principally because they produce quite similar disease states. There are of course definite distinctions between the two, most obviously in the area of systemic effects. In pooling these diseases together for the purposes of this paper, the often thin line between Addison's disease and "acute adrenal crisis" has been set aside in order to create an effective comparative discourse. Acute adrenal crisis refers to the state of collapse often followed swiftly by shock, due to failure of the body's own hormone products (i.e. those made by the body, as opposed to hormone "supplements" prescribed by a medical practitioner).

The purpose of this integrated thesis and research project is to compare the clinical presentations, laboratory findings, and key medical management principles for two endocrine diseases. The first disease discussed is Addison's disease, a condition characterized by adrenocortical insufficiency, and the second is Cushing syndrome, a condition of adrenocortical hyperfunction. Both of these diseases feature alterations in pituitary-adrenal negative feedback pathways (albeit with different primary etiologies) that result in abnormalities in circulating hormones of the hypothalamic-pituitary-adrenal axis. The delineation of such similarities will elucidate a well-rounded portrait of the key features of both disorders. The actual diagnosis and treatment of these diseases is not treated in this paper, as these subjects are beyond the scope of this investigation. Furthermore, while the disease states may be of extracurricular interest, rareness dictates that such topics compel neither our attention nor detailed study here. This paper has some limitations. Firstly, the representation of the diseases is not exhaustive. Instead, a range of characteristics is provided which is considered to be valid for a basic understanding of the disorders. Secondly, as with all papers, the information is likely to have a predetermined cultural slant, depending on the source and the setting.

Comparative study of Addison's disease and Cushing syndrome: Purpose and scope

2. Anatomy and Physiology of the Adrenal Glands

In the body, cortisol makes sure that the cells and tissues get enough energy and nutrition, especially during periods of stress (physical, emotional, trauma, surgery, exercise, infection, or illness). These situations can cause swelling, inflammation, pain, and other symptoms in the body. So, the primary purpose of cortisol is to provide the nutrients and energy needed to heal tissues, fight infection, and help the body function well under stress. In addition, it has a major role in the body's adaptation in stress conditions. It helps the body to reach a balance called homeostasis, where the internal body environment remains stable and functions smoothly, even though there are changes in the exterior bodily or emotional environment. In this situation, cortisol has a catabolic function, which means it facilitates breaking down tissues and fuel storage to use in stressful states. This effect enables the body to identify what tissues need more energy to function, even when the body's energy requirements are the same.

The adrenal glands are two triangular-shaped glands located at the top of both kidneys (Figure 1). The adrenal glands are made of two parts – the adrenal medulla and the adrenal cortex, both of which make important hormones. The adrenal medulla is the inner part of the adrenal gland. When stimulated by the nervous system, the adrenal medulla makes a hormone called adrenaline (also called epinephrine). The adrenal cortex is the outer part of the adrenal gland. It makes a number of hormones. Cortisol is one of the most important and abundant hormones, which is secreted by the zona fasciculata of the adrenal cortex and is one of the glucocorticoids.

2.1. Structure of the Adrenal Glands

The human adrenal glands are endocrine organs consisting of both a cortex and a medulla. The medulla is centrally located within two grooves, but is an embryologically, histologically, functionally, and biochemically different gland. The cortex constitutes about 90% of the gland and is yellow and three times heavier and four times larger than the adrenal medulla. The largest of the two adrenal glands, the right, weighs about 10 g and volume of 10 mL, while the left adrenal gland weighs about 5 g and volume of 5 mL. The adrenal glands are pyramidal in shape, sitting on the superomedial aspect of both kidneys. In humans, the glands are protected by Gerota's fascia and spread 56% over the kidney superomedial aspect. The normal adrenal gland developed into a horseshoe shape during gestation, but regressed to 80% afterwards. The structure of the adrenal glands remains consistent with aging, except for the degree of central fat accumulation and gland atrophy. Inheritance and several external physical factors affect the volume and functions of the adrenal glands. The adrenal cortex consists of three morphologically and hormonally distinct zones, and its structure and functions have been described in detail.

The hormones that maintain homeostasis, like glucocorticoids, mineralocorticoids, and catecholamines, play a crucial role in regulating body temperature, plasma osmolarity, blood volume, and the mechanisms of a fight and flight response. Adrenal gland volume and its mineralocorticoid, cortisol, and catecholamine biosynthesis are regulated by the renin-angiotensin-aldosterone system (RAAS), the hypothalamic-pituitary-adrenocortical (HPA) axis, and the autonomic nervous system. Adrenal blood flow is highly regulated and important to hormone delivery, paracrine systems, adrenocortical function, adrenal mass growth, necrosis, and the responses to various adrenocortical stresses. The structure of the adrenal glands contributing to their function is described here. The adrenal cortex consists of three layers (zona glomerulosa; zona fasciculata; zona reticularis) that produce mineralocorticoids, glucocorticoids, androgens, and estrogen, respectively, that are secreted into the bloodstream.

2.2. Functions of Cortisol

Stress is the sum of the physical and mental reactions we undergo in regard to our environment. When subjected to typical physical, emotional, or oxidative stressors, such as those that might be the result of a real or perceived threat, normal reaction may result in "stress" that agitates the homeostatic status of the animal. Both cats and dogs are known to have selective immunosuppression of the humoral arm during periods of increased cortisol, caused by the activation of T-cells, in addition to lymphostenosis. Steroids, including the glucocorticoids, have not been demonstrated to be lipophilic; however, they have been shown to move readily in some animal models through the blood-brain barrier. It has been found that hepatocytes secrete pro-ideation molecules, growth hormone, and various insulin-like growth factors, as is the case with these hormones, but muscles are the major site for the synthesis of insulin-like growth factors.

Now we can discuss the functionality of the various components of the structure outlined above. Starting with cortisol, which is among the glucocorticoids produced by the zona fasciculata of the adrenal cortex. It is the primary member of a group of metabolically related compounds called glucocorticoids because of their role in influencing glucose metabolism. Cells of most tissues are involved with the reception of glucocorticoids because of the profound metabolic involvement of the hormone. Besides the alterations discussed with regard to glucose and proteometabolism, cortisol stimulates the breakdown of fat, stimulates the production of cholesterol, makes cells more responsive to other hormones involved with lipogenesis in some tissues, conserves blood glucose by the stimulation of muscle to break down proteins, and promotes gluconeogenesis in the liver. In response to stress, the consolidation of glucose as the major energy substrate fuels enhanced muscle function in an acute physiologic manner.

3. Addison's Disease

Cushing syndrome describes the signs and symptoms associated with excessive levels of cortisol. The most common cause of endogenously excessive cortisol is a pituitary adenoma (approximately 70% of patients with Cushing's syndrome). An ectopic corticotropin-releasing hormone (CRH) or adrenocorticotropic hormone (ACTH) secretion from a non-pituitary tumour is the cause in 15% of patients. Bilateral adrenocortical neoplasia accounts for less than 15% of the remaining cases and is usually due to micronodular or macronodular hyperplasia or to a benign adenoma. Other causes of endogenous cortisol excess include bilateral adrenalectomy or accidental adrenal infarction (50% of cases) in which an ACTH-secreting tumour was also resected, and rare causes of hypercortisolism, such as primary pigmented nodular adrenocortical disease, bilateral primary adrenal micronodular hyperplasia and cortisol-producing adrenal tumours in the context of familial neoplasia syndromes. Cushing's disease is three to four times more common in women than in men. A peak incidence of Cushing's disease is found during the 20-40-year age range. It results from excess ACTH production by the pituitary adenoma and has a female-to-male ratio of about 3:1. Approximately 10-15% of affected patients have a macro-adenoma, and 85-90% a micro-adenoma. The higher incidence in women and the higher prevalence of macroadenomas is due to the fact that Cushing's disease is associated with an increase in the ACTH receptor and an overexpression of the corticotrophin-releasing hormone receptor in the pituitary, which causes gland hyperplasia.

Adrenal insufficiency and Addison's disease are often used interchangeably. Primary adrenal insufficiency is referred to as Addison's disease. The most common cause of Addison's disease is autoimmune, and it is more common in women than in men. Destruction of the adrenal glands by autoantibodies is thought to be due to a virus, a unique infecting agent, or a defect in the immune system regulation that allows an immune reaction against the body's adrenal tissue (an autoimmune disease). A history of autoimmune disease in the family increases the risk of disease. Non-autoimmune causes of Addison's disease are infections, e.g. caused by tuberculosis or HIV and adrenal gland cancer or metastases. In congenital adrenal hyperplasia, a genetic defect in the synthesis of adrenal hormones can result in the impaired development of the adrenal cortex. Acute crisis due to excessive stress, e.g. at higher temperatures or illnesses, in addition to a lack of adrenal hormone and aldosterone, can be fatal without immediate treatment. Symptoms and signs in Addison's disease are due to a lack of adrenal hormones and in the case of primary adrenal insufficiency (Addison's disease) also lack of aldosterone. Diagnosis is made by hormone testing and antibody testing. In addition, it is possible to diagnose both morphological and functional adrenal gland changes using imaging tests.

3.1. Causes and Risk Factors

Addison's disease is a chronic condition in which the adrenal glands, which produce 50 steroid hormones, are destroyed by the body's own immune system. This is more common in adults, especially women. The condition is due to damage to the adrenal cortex, the outer part of the adrenal gland. Most of the causes of primary adrenal insufficiency initiate atrophy of the adrenal glands, resulting in an increased release of the pituitary gland hormone adrenocorticotropic hormone (ACTH) in an attempt to stimulate steroid hormone production. Normal adrenal glands cannot increase cortisol secretion significantly in the presence of stress, disease, or injury. Infections are the leading cause, which can occur suddenly or gradually due to chronic tuberculosis, chronic fungal infections, and meningeal malignancies. Other causes include hydraulic bleeding, anticoagulant therapy, and adrenal vein thrombosis. Autoimmune diseases can cause adrenal failure syndrome, such as Waterhouse-Friderichsen and Addison disease. Mitochondrial adrenal disease can develop at any time in childhood or adulthood, with the majority of the cases beginning in the third or the fourth decade of life.

Addison's disease, also called adrenal insufficiency, is a rare and potentially life-threatening disorder caused by deficient adrenal steroid hormone production. In the developed world, 90-95% of cases are caused by autoimmune adrenalitis. The remainder result from infectious adrenalitis, infiltrative processes, and iatrogenic causes, although some cases may be idiopathic. Less common adrenal autoantibodies associated with autoimmune adrenalitis include antibodies to the steroidogenic enzymes side-chain cleavage (SCC: P450scc), 21-hydroxylase (P450c21), steroid 17a-hydroxylase (P450c17), and steroid 21-hydroxylase (P450c21), neither of which correlates with the degree of adrenal failure. Sepsis is the most common cause of acquired primary adrenal insufficiency, which is often reversible.

3.2. Clinical Presentation

Patients with AD can present with a multitude of signs and symptoms, as manifestations of glucocorticoid, mineralocorticoid, adrenal androgen, and other contributed deficiencies including skin hyperpigmentation due to elevated ACTH and MSH. Hypotension and the occasional manifestation of orthostatic hypotension as a result of massive volume contraction and salt depletion secondary to lack of aldosterone and cortisol combine to form one of the cornerstones of AD presentation. The so-called "classic triad" includes weakness, weight loss, and bronze skin pigmentation. However, this clinical triad was only seen in 2.8–10.6% of a random European patient sample and none of Flemish AD patients at diagnosis. Classic findings in patients with GC deficiency comprise chronic fatigue, anorexia, weight loss, and nausea. Patients also report a reduced overall sense of well-being, irritability, reduced ability to concentrate, mild depressive symptoms, disturbed sleep, and subfebrile temperatures. Hyperpigmentation is generally not an early sign and is mainly associated with otherwise unexplained weight loss. Other prominent symptoms of the mineralocorticoid deficiency include hyperkalemia with paresthesias, muscle weakness, and, most commonly, arterial hypotension. However, while these are early presentations in some patients, others have been found to feature normal potassium levels and normal blood pressure upon diagnosis.

According to their respective diseases, Addison and Cushing had experienced both the hypoadrenal and the hyperadrenal clinical consequences of chronic insufficiency of their adrenal cortex. Their clinical signs and symptoms were related to the predominant disturbances of water, mineral, and carbohydrate metabolism then elaborated on by the hormone specialists of their respective times.

4.4. Clinical Presentation

4. Results

4. Cushing Syndrome

Patients who develop salt excess and edema may be asymptomatic, but most will report subjective complaints of "puffiness" or facial swelling as their first more serious complaint. In this situation, overproduction of other steroids, besides hypercortisolism, is classically reported, especially in overt and severe Cushing syndrome. Smaller adenomas, micronodules, and secreting hyperplasia can mimic the hormonal pattern of ectopic ACTH syndrome or Cushing disease, but it is usually a combination of steroid hormonal excess that makes the distinction between eutopic ACTH excess (mainly progressing to cortisol) and non-ACTH mediated steroid excess.

The pathophysiologic changes that occur in Cushing syndrome depend on many variables, including gender, age, environmental influences, which do not attenuate over time, and stage of recovery when treatment is initiated. In adults of both sexes exposed to excessive glucocorticoids, multiple immediate or acute effects have been described. The frontal cortical structures can also be affected by prolonged glucocorticoid exposure. For a discrete overspill effect, edema and swelling of the temporal and frontal lobes, along with the trans-synaptic effect of the tumoral environment, can act as an independent mechanism to cause central nervous system effects, including ataxia, by pressure effects and also attention and memory impairment. These patients are not candidates for quick return of vision or neurological symptoms because the vessels in question feared contain extensive collateral supply, and opening them could produce a catastrophic hypertensive stroke.

Although most of the appreciable daily cortisol production in healthy people is regulated by activation of the hypothalamic-pituitary-adrenal (HPA) axis, this system is "programmed" early in pregnancy after the first trimester, when the placenta increases maternal cortisol binding globulin, thereby decreasing plasma free cortisol. As a result, plasma ACTH levels are decreased, and hyperplasia of the zona fasciculata of the fetal adrenal is minimal. As a result, maternal cortisol levels must increase five to seven-fold for much of pregnancy. Therefore, only excessive fetal or trans-placental cortisol or other stimulating molecules should be able to cause a continuum of cortisol excess from tainting to Cushing syndrome in any parturient.

Cushing syndrome presents with signs and symptoms unique to the individual and is often diagnosed by biochemical testing. Although extensive research has been performed for over 80 years on the pathophysiology of Cushing syndrome, the exact etiology remains unknown. The syndrome itself simply represents end-organ exposure to excessive glucocorticoids (cortisol or other exogenous steroids). Since the cortisol circadian rhythm is impaired in only about a quarter of cases, it is unclear whether loss of the nocturnal nadir of cortisol is a critical component of pathogenesis.

4.1. Etiology and Pathophysiology

Pathophysiology. CS develops following alterations in the HPA axis-mediated feedback control of cortisol release and the loss of the circadian rhythm. Plasma cortisol levels peak early in the morning, and circulatory corticosteroid-binding globulin (CBG), plasma ACTH, and cortisol levels undergo ultradian pulses during the day. The hypothalamus synthesizes corticotropin-releasing hormone (CRH) and vasopressin, which regulate ACTH synthesis. ACTH, in turn, binds to the melanocortin type-2 receptor that is distributed in the zona fasciculata and, to a lesser extent, in the zona reticularis. This event leads to cholesterol ester hydrolysis and ACTH-driven cholesterol import, thereby increasing adrenal steroidogenesis, mainly of cortisol. Both CRH and ACTH secretion are subject to the pulsatile rhythm with periodic appearance and disappearance of secretory bursts occurring in a quadratic pattern.

Etiology. Exogenous or endogenous exposure to glucocorticoids causes Cushing syndrome (CS). The commonest cause of endogenous Cushing syndrome is Cushing disease, which is caused by adrenocorticotropic hormone (ACTH)-secreting pituitary adenomas. The other etiologic factors include ectopic Cushing syndrome, primary adrenal diseases (Cushing syndrome), and familial Cushing syndrome. The most common cause of endogenous hypercortisolemia is ACTH-independent adrenal CS. The most common causes of ACTH-independent CS are adrenocortical adenomas and adrenocortical carcinomas. SCS results from long-term therapy with moderate to high-dose glucocorticoids (GC) in diverse illnesses, but the likelihood of developing SCS is low in any individual treated with GC. Patients with CS may have coexisting autonomous production of androgens or mineralocorticoids leading to overt or subclinical Cushing syndrome as well as androgen or mineralocorticoid excess; they may also have biochemical piggyback phenomena. Most patients with CS are aged 20–50 years.

4.2. Clinical Features

Because the mucinous adenoma alters glucose tolerance, overt diabetes is more common. While it is true that many reports suggest the presence of glucose intolerance in Cushing syndrome, definite evidence to date indicates that these changes are subtler than in the MCA-induced Cushing syndrome. Some degree of hypertension falls within its varying classification. More marked hypertension is seen in those with PSE of Cushing syndrome; electrocardiographic changes with right or complete hypertrophy.

DK wrote an article some time ago summarizing the clinical features of Cushing syndrome. Only a few minor additions have been made to the list since then. The majority of all cases of Cushing syndrome are related to an ACTH-secreting pituitary microadenoma. In early or orange obesity, the centripetal obesity is more marked than in other forms of obesity. The more marked skin changes in patients with Cushing syndrome are purplish striae wider than 1 cm and hypertrichosis. Three-quarters of all patients with Cushing syndrome have acute or chronic weakness. Muscle atrophy is present in one-half of all cases of Cushing syndrome. The large trunk is a common feature in patients with Cushing syndrome. Hypertension is common in patients with Cushing syndrome, and those with PSE of Cushing syndrome verify this fact. More than 40% of adults with Cushing syndrome note some marked emotional upset. Depressive reaction as a major feature of the clinical picture of Cushing syndrome may be reported anywhere from 15 to 80% of all patients.

More recently various forms of hypertension have been described in Cushing syndrome.

5. Diagnosis and Differential Diagnosis

Imaging studies Adrenal computed tomography (CT) or magnetic resonance imaging (MRI) show bilateral adrenal gland atrophy or calcium staining with a TPST of 300 min (about 84% of patients). But in Cushing syndrome, the sensitivity to identify adrenal calcification rises only with a TPST of at least 20 years. Positron emission tomography (PET-CT) or thorium computed tomography show symmetrically diffuse or moderate attenuation with a TPST of 300 min (about 80-85% of patients). In 90% of men with Addison's disease, a pineal gland calcification only detectable by cephalograms at the age of 40 years is present. In Addison disease with postural pressure, the typical meningeal (Leo rigidity, Kernig, Brudzinski, Valsalva signs) and visual (fayret, Delius, Oppenheim, Schirmers test) symptoms combined or not, are pathognomonic, but are not observed in the normotensive patients or only occasionally in the investigating supine hypotensive patients. Although the diagnosis of Addison's disease, as well as Cushing syndrome, is specially nominated by laboratory parameters of primary aldosteronism, a rare case of Addison's disease with hyperaldosteronism has been demonstrated. Several methods are used for confirming the diagnosis of Addison's disease and for differentiating the etiology of adrenal insufficiency: the traditional imaging tests (the monitoring of active renin and the adrenocorticotropic hormone, of the circadian rhythm); measuring the plasma volume and the reactive hyperaemical reserve of plasma volume, the salt test, and the ophthalmodynamometry.

Laboratory tests Adrenal antibodies are present in 20-30% of patients with Addison's disease, which are negative in most cases of Cushing syndrome. Dehydroepiandrosterone (DHEA) and androstenedione serum levels are suppressed in 80-90% of patients with both primary and secondary adrenal insufficiency. They are elevated in about 60-70% of patients with adrenal hyperactivity of Cushing syndrome, but adrenal androgens serum levels are within the normal range in 30-40% of hypophyseal-adrenal adenylate cyclase activating syndrome. Cytomegalovirus seropositive results are less frequent in patients with Cushing syndrome compared to those with Addison's disease. Absolute eosinopenia is characteristic of primary and secondary adrenal insufficiency in up to 75% and 60% of patients, respectively. Innumerable associations or dissociations of the level of 17-OHCS and of 17-KS have been described, with no consensus over any differential diagnoses established by those data. The retromolar pad area of CT/MRI or PET-CT-guided core-needle adrenal biopsy characteristics of small or medium size; thick retroperitoneal fat over the adrenal trace was only present in patients with steatotic adrenal glands compared to those without it.

5.1. Laboratory Tests

Addison's disease is almost always associated with primary hypoadrenalism, and therefore, in all cases except those with ongoing corticosteroid treatment, the basal test is enough to establish the diagnosis: increased plasma ACTH levels, low plasma cortisol levels, and increased plasma renin levels. For a number of reasons and under several conditions, it is possible to perform a synacthen test. It is also possible to assess plasma dehydroepiandrosterone, a precursor of aldosterone derived from the reticular zone (RZ) of the adrenal cortex. Heterogeneous causes of AI do have to be looked for: antibodies (21sOHAb), MRI, adrenocortical antibodies, gammaglutamyltransferase, complete blood count (CBC), G6PD, electrolytes (potassium and phosphate), acid-base status, serum creatinine, serum cortisol, prolactin, adrenocorticotropic hormone (ACTH). It is also important to assess whether the patient presents signs or symptoms of chronic aldosterone deficiency, including diuresis and blood pressure values. Finally, it is important to look for clinical signs of skin hyperpigmentation. Given that a number of conditions could result in hypothyroidism, a CBC and a free thyroxin (fT4) plasma concentration could be useful in order to exclude a rare concomitant primary hypothyroidism.

In the diagnostic procedure, laboratory tests have a key role. The concept of laboratory testing is extensive, including biochemical investigations of blood and byproducts in the urine and other body fluids. Given that there can be no direct measurement of the functions of the adrenal cortex, the laboratory methods make use of the technologies of measuring steroid plasma and steroid urine.

5.2. Imaging Studies

The imaging assessment of the tumor should be performed by an experienced radiologist, and an imaging report should be guided by the indication of the radiologist, who, in turn, also gives hard to read patterns the differential diagnosis. For establishing the best imaging protocol, the recommendations from the latest version of ENDOG-PC should be consulted. Localization of the corticotroph source in CD could be performed by MRI and CT, as reported in one section. One pilot study reported that adrenocortical scintigraphy technique [18F]FDG-PET/MRI Skov showed visually lower uptake of 18F-FDG in the right adrenal both unstimulated SD, and 30 and min after IV administration in dogs with cortisol-related diseases and healthy animals, suggesting good results in identifying changes related to hypercortisolism, even if no significant quantitative differences were detected between affected and control animals.

5.2. Imaging Studies. The diagnostic tests can guide the use of imaging, which may include anatomic and/or functional procedures. Cross-sectional imaging methods (CT or MRI) are used for locating the tumor or ectopic source, and conventional MRI and MR spectroscopy are compared in Section 6. Generally, the best approach is to correlate the presenting syndromes with the possible location and radiological image of the tumor. For example, tests with high ACTH together with the image of an adrenal mass suggest PPNAD, which can also present with an incomplete CD phenotype, with no overt Cushing syndrome.

6. Treatment Approaches

The treatment of Cushing syndrome relies on halting the cause of cortisol excess. There are few pharmacological options to control cortisol excess, most of them are old and mostly osilodrostat is a valid treatment, but of its cost and availability. Bilateral adrenalectomy is considered a safe option, with later need lifelong replacement. Unilateral adrenalectomy could be considered in the rare cases of nodular adrenal disease of an adrenal incidentaloma in patients with Cushing's disease, but data is scarce. Radiation is utilized in patients with persistent CD after bilateral adrenalectomy while food and drug administration (FDA)-approved for patients who cannot undergo bilateral adrenalectomy, it is not approved as part of a combination therapy. More research is needed to define the best approach. And further research is needed to define better non-surgical treatments including POMC and other genetic-based agents.

The therapy in Addison's disease is a substitution of deficient hormones. Daily glucocorticoid supplementation is the mainstay of initial therapy. Oral tablets corresponding to 20-30 mg of hydrocortisone in 2-3 divided doses are recommended, corresponding to the replacement of the morning cortisol rise. Stress dosing is necessary in multiple occasions, including surgeries and dental procedures. Conventional regimes involve 20 mg of hydrocortisone (10 mg twice daily in adults) as the morning (M) dose, 10 mg as the early-afternoon (L) dose and 5-10 mg late-afternoon (D) dose. Modified release hydrocortisone (dose equivalents in glucose:Solu-cortef are 11.1 mg, 5.5 mg, 2.7 mg levels of cortisol) given once daily in the early morning, is the recommended treatment for enabling a physiological cortisol rhythm (high dose M-Cort dose of 20-30 mg) and its use should be encouraged in patients on conventional therapy who are experiencing uncontrolled disease. Fludrocortisone is the DOC with a dose of 0.05-0.2 mg daily. Mineralocorticoid replacement is important for Richter's syndrome and controlling symptoms of aldosterone precursor accumulation (HTN, hypokalaemia, metabolic alkalosis). Sodium supplementation might be necessary, especially in hot conditions. Dehydroepiandrosterone in Addison's patients with lowered libido, but not recommended based on the Predict study.

6.1. Pharmacological Interventions

For pediatric patients with congenital adrenal hyperplasia, current first-line pharmacological intervention is low-dose glucocorticoids aiming to suppress ACTH production, lower adrenal androgen, and prevent further androgen-related damage. The synthetic cortisol analogs exert feedback inhibition on the hypothalamus and pituitary, reducing the amount of endogenous adrenal androgen production and revealing blood pressure effects by decreasing extracellular volume. Biotransformation through 11β-hydroxysteroid dehydrogenase type 2 (11-HSD2) makes prednisolone and dexamethasone inactive or poorly active at the mineralocorticoid receptor, thereby preventing hypertension.

For Addison's disease, medications that replace glucocorticoids and mineralocorticoids are commonly prescribed. The synthetic analogs of cortisol possess a higher affinity for the glucocorticoid and mineralocorticoid receptor compared to hydrocortisone with a longer half-life, which enables a more consistent control of cortisol levels. Types of glucocorticoid replacement therapy include hydrocortisone (Cortef, physiologic replacement), prednisone (Deltasone), prednisolone (Prelone), dexamethasone (Decadron), and methylprednisolone (Medrol, steroid replacement). The dosage is decreased as prednisone is the inactive form of prednisolone with an onset of action of 60 min, and the dosage is the lowest for dexamethasone as it is about 20-30 times more potent than cortisol. Types of mineralocorticoid therapy include fludrocortisone (Florinef, mineralocorticoid replacement). The physiological action of fludrocortisone is similar to those of aldosterone, causing sodium reabsorption in the distal tubules, increasing urinary potassium excretion, stimulating urinary dilution in the kidneys, and indirectly increasing water reabsorption.

The pharmacological interventions utilized within the treatment of both Addison's disease and congenital adrenal hyperplasia aim to replace and/or suppress the excess production of adrenal hormones to restore and maintain hormonal balance.

6.2. Surgical Options

Medical complications that can result from this microscopic surgery include injury to the dura and CSF leak. Hemorrhage, in particular, can occur in 2% to 5% of the cases. In the vast majority, this is self-limiting but can occasionally be fatal. Because the dura has a rich arterial blood supply, secondary to the meninges, direct pressure or a muscle sandwich cannot always achieve hemostasis. If this does not control the bleeding, a combination of muscle, bone wax, and dural sealant can be used successfully. At the University of Virginia, we have had to use the posterior approach in only two of 1000 cases. Necrotizing hypophysitis, diabetes insipidus, and CSF leak can occur after surgery. Central diabetes insipidus results from damage to the hypothalamus or from damage occurring as the pituitary stalk and gland are transsected. Postoperative diabetes insipidus will likely resolve. Rarely, postoperative panhypopituitarism can occur. Additionally, a CSF leak can develop postoperatively, especially if it was not recognized during the original surgery. A post-operative leak can be successfully managed with lumbar drainage and occasional hospital confinement until it resolves. In rare cases, reoperation may become necessary.

Surgical options. The initial therapy for patients who are surgical candidates will be the transsphenoidal approach to a macroadenoma. In some cases, medical therapy can be used to improve the health of a patient who is not a surgical candidate. Definitive surgery can treat the acute, chronic effects of hypersecretion as well as the mass effect of the tumor. It should be done by a pituitary surgeon with an expertise in both the pathology and the surgical approach. Transsphenoidal surgery for the resection of the ACTH-producing adenoma leads to resolution or transient amelioration of the hypercortisolemia in 60 to 90% of the cases. The remission rate is dependent on preceding operating therapy. Complicating factors include the size and extension of the adenoma, which improve when the adenoma is primary through the or closely related to the inferior part of the gland. Improved outcomes have also been reported in institutions in which the surgeons are pituitary endocrinology trained. Decreasing the ACTH levels without altering cortisol values is a predictor of good outcome; therefore, in intraoperative monitoring, the plasma cortisol level at corticotropin injection seems a good marker at the end of the removal. Postoperative cortisol levels are checked at 07:00 AM in these early days. Early hypocorticism is checked and corrected with hydrocortisone, and a modified examination with the prolonged low-dose corticotropin test changes to determine adrenal function.

7. Prognosis and Complications

The most serious complication is adrenal crisis, which may correspond to the clinical debut or new diagnosis of the disease. Acute adrenal crisis is a life-threatening condition that is characterized by hypotension, hypovolemic shock, fever, altered consciousness, muscle weakness, hyperkalemia or hyponatremia, and vomiting. Almost all of the untreated patients (90%) with Addison's disease are expected to be admitted to the hospital with an adrenal crisis. Some patients with Addison's disease may have an adrenal crisis which is not as acute because of progressive onset. The admission diagnosis of Addison's disease in the hospital from an adrenal crisis is usually more difficult and may be delayed, posing the patient at a greater risk of collapse, arrhythmias, and eventually death. Palmieri et al. admit that unrecognized primary adrenal failure when it's the cause was found in 1.6% of cases. Immunologic Addison's disease is associated with celiac disease. Adrenal autoantibodies are online detected in about 23-67% of the patients. Coercive should be suspected. Other complications include a low mood, fatigue, menstrual system disorder, decreased bone density, weight loss, and gastrointestinal symptoms, particularly in autoimmune adrenalitis. This systemic disorder may be associated with changes in the skin, with generalized hyperpigmentation observed mainly in exposed areas. Sequent regression to a coma may maintenance requirement of glucocorticoids in patients with autoimmune Addison's disease. Doses of 25-50 mg of prednisolone appear to reduce blood concentrations of 17-azar by 50 to 60% and should be used in association maintenance treatment with increasing nossa zod. A small percentage of patients with Addison's or premature ovarian failure who were pregnant have reading a combined decrease in aldosterone and hypothalamic disease with defivult women rate pregnancy. For most of these women, pregnancy is considered to be at high risk, accrues in conjunction with a multidisciplinary team and advice. Women may have serious complications (most patients spontaneous abortion under 30% of diagnosed pregnancies) and only a reduced number of full-term women are delivered from 20% to 40%. In pregnancy, because of fluid and electrolyte balance issues. A successful pregnancy in women with Addison's disease demonstrates the recovery in stress hormonal response in the third trimester of pregnancy and reduced glucocorticoid requirements. In summary, although Addison's disease is primarily a chronic condition, it may have more serious complications that require accident attention and treatment. It is mainly linked with an increased risk of adrenal crisis. Maintaining regular contact with a team of professionals is encouraged in the diagnosis and follow-up cases.

Complications of Addison's Disease

Addison's disease is chronic and requires lifelong replacement therapy with glucocorticoid and mineralocorticoid. Patients can have a normal lifespan if appropriately treated. An adequate dose of hydrocortisone is proposed to be 3/4 of the daily physiological cortisol production, divided into two-thirds in the morning and one-third in the evening to avoid over-replacement and excess of glucocorticoids. Stress: Illness, intercurrent infections, and other stressful situations may increase glucocorticoid replacement necessary. Patients with Addison's disease should be taught to vary the dose according to the situation (the "sick-day rules"). A crisis may appear when patients do not increase the glucocorticoid dose during stress, which can be life-threatening.

Prognosis: Addison's Disease

8. Research and Future Directions

In conclusion, a comparison between Addison's disease and Cushing syndrome is interesting, since they are both caused by an excessive or an obviated cortisol production, although being a real opposite condition. The most outstanding aspect in the comparison is the different involvement of the endocrine glands, including the relative hormone's impregnation in tissues and cells. Treatment of these disorders is mainly driven by targeting the highest point of the hormone secretion. A pitfall to be taken into account is when the topographical root of the pathological hormone secretion has been removed, and the current patient's conditions are encompassed more by the tissue response to previous "over stimulation," than from the remaining over raised hormone's secretion. Despite resolving the diseased metabolism condition, it is time for "venting the lung". Summing up, the hormones at the clinical, metabolic, and physic-social effects and the intrinsic/overall situation of the body can be considered an engineered tot. What remains unclear is the order of priority between the "metabolic" restoration and the removal of the body's bedsores persisting over time. More recently, besides the aforementioned research and freeways, a further prospective aim should be to investigate cosmetics' change with the use of high-sensitive cortisol measurement in a very large cohort of PCOS patients.

Research for this issue is still active and future research might include the following aspects. A worldwide survey to approach the attitudes of the endocrine societies and any individual endocrinologist to select the best assay used for the diagnosis of Addison's disease. A further step should be to clarify whether cortisol plasma measurement or the ACTH measurement can be negotiated in the era of the introduction of the high-sensitive cortisol assay. The characteristics of patients who are inadequately operated on for Cushing syndrome and the peculiarities of the centers or surgeons with unduly lower success rates in remission compared with the state of the art response rates. Lastly, more evidence might be added about the pathways and involved cells inducing the persistent metabolic abnormalities in the different forms of hypercortisolism.

Made in United States
Orlando, FL
31 December 2024

56734845R00046